A Vaccine - Friendly Guide

For

Parenting

A Practical Approach for Building Stronger Families through informed wellness, and unlocking Health Potential.

Carmen R. Brown

<u>TABLE OF CONTENT</u>

Introduction

Welcome to "A Vaccine-Friendly Guide for Parenting: A Practical Approach for Building Stronger Families through Informed Wellness, and Unlocking Health Potential." This book aims to be your comprehensive guide in navigating the complex and often confusing world of vaccines, providing clear and evidence-based information to help you make the best health decisions for your family.

In today's world, parents face a deluge of information about vaccines, much of which is contradictory and confusing. The goal of this book is to cut through the noise and present factual, balanced, and accessible information about vaccines. By understanding the science behind vaccines and the benefits they offer, you can make informed decisions that protect your child's health and contribute to the well-being of your community.

Parenting is a journey filled with joy, challenges, and responsibilities. Ensuring your child's health and safety is one of the most important responsibilities you have. Vaccines are a critical tool in this effort, protecting against diseases that can cause serious illness or even death. However, the topic of vaccination can be fraught with fear and misinformation, leading to uncertainty and hesitation among parents. This book seeks to alleviate those fears by providing reliable information and practical advice.

This book is not about telling you what to do. Instead, it aims to empower you with knowledge so that you can make the best decisions for your child and your family. Whether you are a new parent, a seasoned caregiver, or simply someone who wants to understand more about vaccines, this guide is designed to be a valuable resource.

Understanding the science behind vaccines is crucial for making informed decisions. Vaccines work by stimulating the immune system to recognize and fight specific pathogens, such as viruses or bacteria, without causing the disease itself. This process involves introducing a harmless component of the pathogen, such as a protein or a weakened form, which trains the immune system to respond effectively if exposed to the actual disease in the future.

The development and testing of vaccines are rigorous processes that ensure their safety and efficacy. Before a vaccine is approved for public use, it undergoes extensive clinical trials involving thousands of participants. These trials assess not only the vaccine's effectiveness in preventing disease but also its safety profile. Once approved, vaccines continue to be monitored for any rare side effects through robust surveillance systems.

Despite the overwhelming evidence supporting the safety and effectiveness of vaccines, misinformation and myths persist. Common myths, such as vaccines causing autism or overwhelming the immune system, have been thoroughly debunked by scientific research. Understanding the origins of these myths and the evidence against them can help alleviate fears and build confidence in vaccination.

A key aspect of a vaccine-friendly approach is building a trusting relationship with healthcare providers. Pediatricians, family doctors, and nurses are invaluable partners in your child's health care. They have the training and experience to provide you with accurate information about vaccines and can help address any concerns or questions you may have.

Trust is built through open communication. Don't hesitate to ask your healthcare provider about the vaccines recommended for your child. Inquire about the benefits, possible side effects, and the diseases they prevent. A good healthcare provider will take the time to listen to your concerns, provide thorough explanations, and respect your role in making decisions for your family.

One of the fundamental principles of vaccination is herd immunity. Herd immunity occurs when a significant portion of a population is immune to a disease, either through vaccination or previous infection, thereby providing indirect protection to those who are not immune. This is particularly important for individuals who cannot be vaccinated due to medical reasons, such as allergies or weakened immune systems.

A vaccine-friendly parent understands the role of community in health and recognizes the collective responsibility to protect vulnerable populations. By vaccinating your child, you are not only safeguarding their health but also contributing to the overall health of your community. This sense of collective responsibility fosters a stronger, healthier society.

A vaccine-friendly approach to parenting is not limited to vaccination alone. It encompasses a broader perspective on health and wellness. This means considering factors such as nutrition, physical activity, mental health, and a supportive environment in promoting overall well-being.

Vaccines are a crucial component of preventive health care, but they are not the only factor in maintaining good health. A balanced diet rich in nutrients, regular physical activity, adequate sleep, and mental health support all contribute to a strong immune system and overall wellness. By adopting a holistic approach to health, you can create a foundation for your child's long-term well-being.

In summary, a vaccine-friendly approach to parenting involves making health decisions based on accurate information, scientific evidence, and a holistic understanding of wellness. It means being informed, thoughtful, and proactive in your family's health care. By educating yourself about vaccines, building trust with healthcare providers, understanding the science, addressing concerns and misconceptions, and considering the broader context of health and wellness, you can make informed decisions that protect your child's health and contribute to the well-being of your community.

Welcome to this journey of informed wellness and stronger families.

Chapter 1: Understanding Vaccines

What Are Vaccines?

Vaccines are biological preparations designed to provide immunity to a particular infectious disease. They contain agents that resemble a disease-causing microorganism and are often made from weakened or killed forms of the microbe, its toxins, or one of its surface proteins. The primary purpose of a vaccine is to stimulate the body's immune system to recognize the agent as a threat, destroy it, and keep a record of it so that the immune system can more easily recognize and destroy any of these microorganisms it encounters later.

The concept of vaccination dates back to the late 18th century when Edward Jenner developed the smallpox vaccine. Jenner observed that milkmaids who had contracted cowpox, a less severe disease, did not get smallpox. By deliberately infecting a boy with cowpox and later exposing him to smallpox, Jenner demonstrated that the boy was immune to smallpox. This groundbreaking work laid the foundation for modern immunology and the development of vaccines.

Vaccines have since become one of the most effective tools in public health. They have led to the eradication of smallpox, the near-eradication of polio, and significant reductions in diseases such as measles, diphtheria, pertussis (whooping cough), and many others. By preventing infectious diseases, vaccines save millions of lives every year and reduce the burden of disease on individuals and healthcare systems.

How Vaccines Work

To understand how vaccines work, it is essential to have a basic understanding of the immune system. The immune system is the body's defense mechanism against infections and other foreign invaders. It consists of various cells and proteins that identify and eliminate pathogens, such as bacteria, viruses, fungi, and parasites.

When a pathogen enters the body, the immune system mounts a response to eliminate it. This response involves two main components: the innate immune response and the adaptive immune response.

1. **Innate Immune Response**: The innate immune response is the body's first line of defense and acts quickly to identify and eliminate pathogens. It involves physical barriers (such as the skin and

mucous membranes), immune cells (such as macrophages and neutrophils), and proteins (such as cytokines) that recognize and destroy invaders.

2. **Adaptive Immune Response**: If the innate immune response is not sufficient to eliminate the pathogen, the adaptive immune response is activated. This response is more specific and involves the activation of lymphocytes (B cells and T cells) that recognize specific components of the pathogen, called antigens. B cells produce antibodies that bind to and neutralize the pathogen, while T cells kill infected cells and help regulate the immune response.

The adaptive immune response has a memory component, meaning that once the immune system has encountered a particular pathogen, it can respond more quickly and effectively upon subsequent exposures. This is the principle behind vaccination.

Vaccines work by mimicking a natural infection without causing disease. They introduce antigens (such as proteins or polysaccharides) from the pathogen into the body, which stimulates the adaptive immune response. This exposure leads to the production of memory cells, which "remember" the pathogen and provide long-lasting immunity. When the vaccinated individual is later exposed to the actual pathogen, their immune system can quickly recognize and eliminate it, preventing illness.

There are several key steps in how vaccines stimulate the immune system:

1. **Antigen Presentation**: The vaccine contains antigens from the pathogen, which are recognized by antigen-presenting cells (APCs) in the body. These APCs, such as dendritic cells, process the antigens and present them on their surface to other immune cells.
2. **Activation of T Cells**: The presented antigens activate T cells, which play a crucial role in coordinating the immune response. Helper T cells (CD4+ T cells) activate B cells and cytotoxic T cells (CD8+ T cells). Cytotoxic T cells kill infected cells, while helper T cells release cytokines that enhance the immune response.
3. **Activation of B Cells**: B cells are activated by the antigens and helper T cells. Activated B cells differentiate into plasma cells, which produce antibodies specific to the antigens. These antibodies bind to the pathogen, neutralizing it

and marking it for destruction by other immune cells.

4. **Formation of Memory Cells**: Some of the activated B cells and T cells become memory cells, which remain in the body for years or even decades. These memory cells provide long-term immunity by rapidly responding to future exposures to the pathogen.

Types of Vaccines and Their Ingredients

Vaccines can be classified into several types based on their composition and the way they stimulate the immune system. Each type of vaccine has its advantages and limitations, and the choice of vaccine depends on various factors, including the nature of the pathogen, the desired immune response, and safety considerations.

1. **Live Attenuated Vaccines**: Live attenuated vaccines contain live but weakened (attenuated) forms of the pathogen. These vaccines closely mimic a natural infection and usually provide long-lasting immunity with one or two doses. Examples include the measles, mumps, and rubella (MMR) vaccine and the oral polio vaccine (OPV).

- **Advantages**: Strong and long-lasting immune response, usually requiring fewer doses.
- **Limitations**: Not suitable for immunocompromised individuals, risk of reversion to a virulent form (rare).

2. **Inactivated (Killed) Vaccines**: Inactivated vaccines contain pathogens that have been killed or inactivated by heat, chemicals, or radiation. These vaccines cannot cause disease but still stimulate an immune response. Examples include the inactivated polio vaccine (IPV) and the hepatitis A vaccine.

   - **Advantages**: Safe for immunocompromised individuals, no risk of reversion to a virulent form.
   - **Limitations**: Generally, require multiple doses and booster shots to maintain immunity.

3. **Subunit, Recombinant, and Conjugate Vaccines**: These vaccines contain only specific parts of the pathogen, such as proteins or polysaccharides, rather than the whole pathogen. Subunit vaccines include the hepatitis B vaccine and the human papillomavirus (HPV) vaccine. Recombinant vaccines are produced using genetic engineering techniques, and conjugate vaccines link polysaccharides to proteins to enhance the immune

response, such as the Haemophilus influenzae type b (Hib) vaccine.

- **Advantages**: Focused immune response to key antigens, safe for immunocompromised individuals.
- **Limitations**: May require adjuvants (substances that enhance the immune response) and multiple doses.

4. **Toxoid Vaccines**: Toxoid vaccines contain inactivated toxins (toxoids) produced by the pathogen. These vaccines target the toxins rather than the pathogen itself. Examples include the diphtheria and tetanus vaccines.

- **Advantages**: Effective against toxin-mediated diseases, stable and safe.
- **Limitations**: May require booster shots to maintain immunity.

5. **Messenger RNA (mRNA) Vaccines**: mRNA vaccines use a small piece of genetic material (mRNA) that instructs cells to produce a protein from the pathogen, which then stimulates an immune response. The COVID-19 vaccines developed by Pfizer-BioNTech and Moderna are examples of mRNA vaccines.

- **Advantages**: Rapid development and production, strong immune response.

- **Limitations**: Require cold storage, potential for short-term side effects.

6. **Viral Vector Vaccines**: Viral vector vaccines use a modified virus (not the pathogen) to deliver genetic material from the pathogen into cells, prompting an immune response. The COVID-19 vaccines developed by Johnson & Johnson and AstraZeneca are examples of viral vector vaccines.
   - **Advantages**: Strong immune response, stable at refrigerator temperatures.
   - **Limitations**: Pre-existing immunity to the vector virus may reduce effectiveness.

Vaccine Ingredients

Vaccines contain various ingredients that contribute to their safety and effectiveness. Understanding these ingredients can help alleviate concerns and provide clarity on how vaccines work.

1. **Antigens**: The active component of the vaccine, which stimulates the immune response. Antigens can be proteins, polysaccharides, or genetic material from the pathogen.
2. **Adjuvants**: Substances added to vaccines to enhance the immune response. Common adjuvants include aluminum salts (e.g., aluminum

hydroxide, aluminum phosphate), which boost the body's response to the antigens.

3. **Stabilizers**: Ingredients that maintain the stability and potency of the vaccine during storage and transportation. Stabilizers can include sugars (e.g., sucrose, lactose), proteins (e.g., gelatin), and amino acids (e.g., glycine).

4. **Preservatives**: Substances that prevent contamination by bacteria or fungi in multi-dose vaccine vials. Thimerosal, a mercury-based preservative, has been used in some vaccines, though it has been largely phased out in favor of other preservatives.

5. **Dilutants**: Sterile liquids used to dilute a vaccine to the correct concentration. Common diluents include sterile water or saline solution.

6. **Residuals**: Trace amounts of substances used in the manufacturing process, such as antibiotics (to prevent bacterial contamination during production), egg proteins (in some flu vaccines), or formaldehyde (used to inactivate pathogens or toxins).

It's important to note that the amounts of these ingredients in vaccines are carefully controlled and rigorously tested to ensure safety and efficacy. Regulatory agencies such as the U.S. Food and Drug

Administration (FDA), the European Medicines Agency (EMA), and the World Health Organization (WHO) oversee the approval and monitoring of vaccines to ensure they meet stringent safety standards.

Understanding vaccines involves recognizing their critical role in public health, how they work to protect against infectious diseases, and the different types of vaccines available. By simulating a natural infection, vaccines train the immune system to recognize and respond to pathogens without causing disease, providing long-lasting immunity.

The various types of vaccines—live attenuated, inactivated, subunit, recombinant, conjugate, toxoid, mRNA, and viral vector—each have unique advantages and limitations, making them suitable for different diseases and populations. The ingredients in vaccines, including antigens, adjuvants, stabilizers, preservatives, diluents, and residuals, are carefully selected and tested to ensure safety and effectiveness.

As a parent, understanding these fundamental aspects of vaccines empowers you to make informed decisions about your child's health. Vaccines are a vital component of preventive health care, protecting individuals and communities from infectious diseases and contributing to the overall well-being of society. By choosing to vaccinate, you are taking an important step in building a healthier future for your child and for generations to come.

Chapter 2: Building Stronger Families

Importance of Family Health and Wellness

The health and wellness of a family are foundational to its strength and happiness. A family's well-being affects every aspect of life, from daily routines to long-term goals and aspirations. In this chapter, we will explore why family health is so critical and how it contributes to the overall strength of the family unit.

Health is often defined as the absence of disease, but it is much more comprehensive. True wellness encompasses physical, mental, emotional, and social well-being. When a family prioritizes wellness, it creates an environment where each member can thrive and reach their full potential.

1. **Physical Health**:
   - **Disease Prevention**: Good physical health practices, such as regular exercise, balanced nutrition, and adequate sleep, play a crucial role in preventing diseases. Regular medical check-ups and vaccinations are also essential in keeping diseases at bay.
   - **Increased Longevity**: Healthy lifestyle choices contribute to increased longevity. Families that

engage in regular physical activities and maintain healthy diets tend to have longer, more fulfilling lives.

- **Enhanced Energy Levels**: Physical health boosts energy levels, enabling family members to participate actively in daily activities, work, and play.

2. **Mental Health**:

- **Stress Reduction**: Mental health is vital for managing stress. A supportive family environment can help members cope with stress more effectively, reducing the risk of mental health issues such as anxiety and depression.
- **Cognitive Function**: Good mental health supports cognitive function, including memory, decision-making, and problem-solving skills. This is especially important for children as they grow and learn.

3. **Emotional Health**:

- **Emotional Resilience**: Families that prioritize emotional health foster resilience. Emotional resilience is the ability to bounce back from adversity, maintain positive relationships, and manage emotions effectively.
- **Positive Relationships**: Emotional health is the cornerstone of positive relationships. Open

communication, empathy, and understanding within the family build strong bonds and a supportive network.

4. **Social Health**:

- **Community Engagement**: Social health involves being part of a community. Families that engage with their community build a support system that can provide assistance and a sense of belonging.
- **Healthy Social Interactions**: Healthy social interactions, both within the family and with others, promote a sense of well-being and connectedness.

The importance of family health and wellness cannot be overstated. It is the foundation upon which families build their lives. When families prioritize health and wellness, they create an environment that supports growth, happiness, and resilience.

Creating a Healthy Home Environment

Creating a healthy home environment is essential for promoting the overall well-being of the family. A healthy home environment encompasses physical, mental, and emotional aspects. Here are several key components and practical steps to achieve this:

1. **Nutrition and Diet**:
   - **Balanced Meals**: Ensure that meals are balanced and nutritious. Include a variety of fruits, vegetables, whole grains, lean proteins, and healthy fats in your family's diet. Avoid processed foods and excessive sugar.
   - **Meal Planning**: Plan meals ahead of time to ensure nutritional balance and to avoid the temptation of unhealthy fast food. Involve family members in meal planning and preparation to encourage healthy eating habits.
   - **Hydration**: Encourage family members to drink plenty of water throughout the day. Limit sugary drinks and sodas.
2. **Physical Activity**:
   - **Regular Exercise**: Promote regular physical activity by incorporating it into daily routines. Family walks, bike rides, and outdoor play can be enjoyable ways to stay active together.
   - **Limit Screen Time**: Set limits on screen time for both children and adults. Encourage physical activities and hobbies that do not involve screens.
   - **Create an Active Environment**: Design your home environment to encourage physical activity. Have sports equipment, bicycles, and outdoor play items readily available.

3. **Mental and Emotional Well-being**:
   - **Open Communication**: Foster an environment of open communication where family members feel comfortable expressing their thoughts and emotions. Regular family meetings can be a good platform for discussions.
   - **Stress Management**: Teach and practice stress management techniques such as mindfulness, meditation, and deep breathing exercises. Encourage hobbies and activities that promote relaxation.
   - **Emotional Support**: Provide emotional support to each family member. Be attentive, listen actively, and show empathy. Recognize and celebrate achievements, both big and small.
4. **Healthy Sleep Habits**:
   - **Consistent Sleep Schedule**: Establish a consistent sleep schedule for all family members. Consistent bedtimes and wake-up times help regulate the body's internal clock.
   - **Sleep Environment**: Create a sleep-friendly environment with comfortable bedding, a dark room, and a cool temperature. Limit noise and distractions in the bedroom.
   - **Screen Time Before Bed**: Reduce screen time before bed as the blue light emitted by screens

can interfere with sleep. Encourage reading or other relaxing activities instead.

5. **Hygiene and Cleanliness**:
   - **Regular Cleaning**: Maintain a clean and organized home environment. Regular cleaning reduces allergens, bacteria, and other health hazards.
   - **Hand Hygiene**: Teach and practice proper hand hygiene, especially before meals and after using the restroom. Good hand hygiene helps prevent the spread of germs.
   - **Safe Environment**: Ensure that the home environment is safe. Childproof areas to prevent accidents, keep hazardous substances out of reach, and ensure that smoke detectors and carbon monoxide detectors are functioning.

6. **Healthy Relationships**:
   - **Quality Time**: Spend quality time together as a family. Shared activities, meals, and traditions strengthen family bonds.
   - **Conflict Resolution**: Teach and practice healthy conflict resolution skills. Address conflicts promptly and constructively.
   - **Supportive Network**: Build and maintain a supportive network of friends, extended family, and community members. A strong support

network provides emotional and practical assistance when needed.

7. **Education and Learning**:
   - **Lifelong Learning**: Promote a culture of lifelong learning. Encourage reading, curiosity, and the pursuit of knowledge.
   - **Educational Support**: Support children's education by being involved in their school activities, helping with homework, and encouraging a love of learning.
   - **Skill Development**: Provide opportunities for family members to develop new skills and hobbies. This can include activities such as cooking, gardening, or playing a musical instrument.

8. **Environmental Health**:
   - **Reduce Toxins**: Minimize exposure to toxins in the home by using natural cleaning products, reducing plastic use, and avoiding products with harmful chemicals.
   - **Indoor Air Quality**: Improve indoor air quality by ventilating the home, using air purifiers, and keeping indoor plants.
   - **Sustainable Practices**: Adopt sustainable practices such as recycling, conserving water, and

reducing energy consumption. Teach children the importance of environmental stewardship.

By focusing on these key components, you can create a home environment that supports the health and wellness of every family member. A healthy home environment is a place where family members feel safe, supported, and empowered to live their best lives.

The health and wellness of a family are paramount to its strength and happiness. Prioritizing physical, mental, emotional, and social health creates a foundation for a thriving family. By implementing practical steps to create a healthy home environment, you can ensure that your family is well-equipped to face life's challenges and enjoy its many joys.

Creating a healthy home environment is an ongoing process that requires commitment and effort from all family members. It is about making conscious choices that promote well-being and foster a supportive and loving atmosphere. By doing so, you are investing in the long-term health and happiness of your family, building a strong foundation for the future.

Chapter 3: The Vaccine-Friendly Approach

Overview of the Vaccine-Friendly Plan

A vaccine-friendly approach to parenting emphasizes informed decision-making, trust in scientific evidence, and a holistic view of health and wellness. This approach is grounded in understanding the benefits and potential risks of vaccines, building strong relationships with healthcare providers, and fostering a community mindset that recognizes the collective responsibility to protect public health. The goal is not only to ensure the health and safety of your children but also to contribute to the overall well-being of society.

Informed Decision-Making

Informed decision-making is the cornerstone of a vaccine-friendly approach. This means parents take an active role in understanding vaccines, how they work, their benefits, and potential side effects. Knowledge empowers parents to make confident choices that are in the best interest of their children and the community.

To be truly informed, parents should seek information from credible sources. These include healthcare providers, peer-reviewed scientific journals, and reputable health organizations like the Centers for

Disease Control and Prevention (CDC), the World Health Organization (WHO), and the American Academy of Pediatrics (AAP). It's also important to be wary of misinformation spread through social media and non-scientific sources.

Understanding Vaccines

Vaccines are biological preparations that provide immunity to specific infectious diseases. They work by mimicking disease agents, such as bacteria or viruses, without causing illness. This process trains the immune system to recognize and fight the actual pathogen if exposed in the future. Understanding this basic mechanism helps demystify vaccines and underscores their role in preventing diseases.

The Importance of Vaccination Schedules

Vaccination schedules are designed to provide immunity at the most appropriate times in a child's development. Following these schedules ensures that children are protected when they are most vulnerable to certain diseases. Delaying or skipping vaccines can leave children exposed to preventable illnesses and can disrupt herd immunity, putting the broader community at risk.

Healthcare providers are invaluable resources for understanding and following vaccination schedules. They can provide personalized recommendations based on a child's health history and ensure that vaccinations are administered safely and effectively.

Building Trust with Healthcare Providers

A trusting relationship with healthcare providers is crucial for a vaccine-friendly approach. Pediatricians, family doctors, and nurses play a vital role in guiding parents through vaccination decisions. Open communication, respect, and collaboration with healthcare providers help build this trust.

Parents should feel comfortable asking questions and expressing concerns about vaccines. A good healthcare provider will listen attentively, provide clear and accurate information, and address any fears or misconceptions. This collaborative approach ensures that parents feel supported and confident in their decisions.

Community and Herd Immunity

Herd immunity occurs when a significant portion of a population becomes immune to a disease, either through vaccination or previous infection, thereby providing indirect protection to those who are not immune. This concept is fundamental to public health as it helps protect vulnerable individuals, such as those who cannot be vaccinated due to medical reasons.

By vaccinating your child, you are not only protecting them but also contributing to the health and safety of your community. This collective responsibility fosters a sense of solidarity and mutual care, essential components of a strong, healthy society.

Benefits of Informed Wellness in Parenting

Informed wellness is about making health decisions based on accurate information and a holistic understanding of wellness. This approach offers numerous benefits, enhancing the health and well-being of both children and parents.

Physical Health Benefits

Vaccines play a crucial role in preventing serious diseases such as measles, mumps, rubella, polio, and whooping cough. These diseases can cause severe complications, long-term health issues, and even death. By following recommended vaccination schedules, parents can protect their children from these risks.

Beyond vaccinations, informed wellness also encompasses other aspects of physical health, such as nutrition, exercise, and sleep. A balanced diet rich in essential nutrients supports the immune system and overall health. Regular physical activity helps maintain a healthy weight, reduces the risk of chronic diseases, and promotes mental well-being. Adequate sleep is essential for growth, cognitive development, and emotional regulation in children.

Mental and Emotional Well-being

Informed wellness also positively impacts mental and emotional health. Parents who are confident in their health decisions tend to experience less anxiety and stress. This confidence comes from understanding the benefits and risks associated with vaccines and other health interventions.

Children benefit from the emotional stability of their parents. When parents are well-informed and less anxious, they can provide a more supportive and reassuring environment for their children. This stable environment is crucial for the emotional development and well-being of children.

Building Resilience

A vaccine-friendly approach helps build resilience in families. Resilience is the ability to adapt and thrive in the face of challenges and adversity. By making informed health decisions, parents can better navigate the complexities of parenting and health care.

Informed wellness encourages proactive health practices, such as regular check-ups, preventive care, and healthy lifestyle choices. These practices help prevent illnesses, manage health conditions effectively, and promote long-term well-being. Resilient families are better equipped to handle health challenges and maintain a high quality of life.

Community Health and Social Responsibility

Informed wellness extends beyond individual and family health to community health. By vaccinating their children, parents contribute to herd immunity, protecting vulnerable individuals who cannot be vaccinated. This collective action demonstrates social responsibility and care for others.

Community health benefits also include reduced healthcare costs and less strain on healthcare systems. Preventing disease through vaccination and informed wellness practices helps reduce the incidence of outbreaks, hospitalizations, and long-term health complications. This, in turn, frees up resources for other critical health needs and improves the overall efficiency of healthcare systems.

Encouraging Critical Thinking and Lifelong Learning

Informed wellness fosters a culture of critical thinking and lifelong learning. Parents who prioritize accurate information and evidence-based practices model these values for their children. This encourages children to develop critical thinking skills and a curiosity for learning, which are essential for their future success.

By staying informed about health and wellness, parents can adapt to new information and changing health recommendations. This flexibility and openness to learning ensure that families remain resilient and well-prepared for future health challenges.

Practical Strategies for Informed Wellness

Implementing a vaccine-friendly and informed wellness approach requires practical strategies and proactive steps. Here are some tips to help parents navigate this journey:

1. **Educate Yourself**: Continuously seek out accurate information about vaccines, health, and wellness. Use reputable sources and stay updated on the latest research and recommendations.
2. **Communicate Openly**: Foster open communication with healthcare providers. Ask questions, express concerns, and seek their guidance in making health decisions.
3. **Prioritize Preventive Care**: Follow recommended vaccination schedules and preventive care practices. Regular check-ups and screenings help detect health issues early and ensure timely interventions.
4. **Adopt a Holistic Approach**: Consider all aspects of health, including nutrition, physical activity, sleep, and mental well-being. A balanced and holistic approach promotes overall health and resilience.
5. **Build a Support Network**: Connect with other parents, community groups, and support organizations. Sharing experiences and knowledge can provide valuable support and encouragement.
6. **Stay Informed and Flexible**: Health recommendations and information can evolve.

Stay informed and be open to adapting your practices based on new evidence and guidance.

7. **Promote Critical Thinking**: Encourage your children to ask questions, seek information, and think critically. This fosters a lifelong love of learning and a proactive approach to health and wellness.

A vaccine-friendly approach to parenting is about more than just following vaccination schedules. It's about making informed decisions based on accurate information, building trust with healthcare providers, and adopting a holistic view of health and wellness. This approach offers numerous benefits, including enhanced physical health, mental and emotional well-being, resilience, and a sense of social responsibility.

By prioritizing informed wellness, parents can ensure the health and safety of their children, contribute to the well-being of their community, and foster a culture of critical thinking and lifelong learning. This comprehensive approach empowers families to thrive and unlocks their full health potential.

Welcome to the journey of informed wellness and stronger families. Together, we can create a healthier, happier future for our children and communities.

Chapter 4: Pregnancy and Childbirth

Preparing for a Healthy Pregnancy

Preparing for a healthy pregnancy is one of the most important steps a woman can take for the health of her future child. This preparation starts long before conception and involves a holistic approach to health and wellness. Here, we will explore the various aspects of preparing for a healthy pregnancy, from physical health to mental well-being, and provide practical advice to help prospective parents embark on this journey with confidence.

Physical Health

1. Preconception Checkup: The journey to a healthy pregnancy begins with a visit to your healthcare provider for a preconception checkup. This visit allows you to discuss your plans and receive personalized advice based on your health history. Your provider may recommend certain tests or screenings to ensure you are in optimal health before conceiving.

2. Nutrition: A balanced diet is crucial for reproductive health. Focus on consuming a variety of nutrient-dense foods, including fruits, vegetables, whole grains, lean proteins, and healthy fats. Key nutrients for preconception include:

- **Folic Acid:** Essential for preventing neural tube defects. Aim for at least 400 micrograms daily, either through diet or supplements.
- **Iron:** Supports the increase in blood volume and prevents anemia. Include iron-rich foods such as lean meats, beans, and spinach.
- **Calcium:** Important for bone health. Dairy products, leafy greens, and fortified foods are good sources.
- **Omega-3 Fatty Acids:** Beneficial for brain and eye development. Include fatty fish like salmon, walnuts, and flaxseeds.

3. Healthy Weight: Achieving and maintaining a healthy weight before pregnancy can reduce the risk of complications. Both underweight and overweight individuals may face challenges. Consult your healthcare provider for guidance on reaching a healthy weight.

4. Exercise: Regular physical activity is beneficial for overall health and can improve fertility. Aim for at least 150 minutes of moderate-intensity exercise per week. Activities such as walking, swimming, and yoga are excellent choices. Avoid high-impact or risky sports that could lead to injury.

5. Avoiding Harmful Substances: Eliminate the use of tobacco, alcohol, and recreational drugs. These substances can negatively impact fertility and the health of a developing fetus. If you need help quitting, seek support from your healthcare provider.

6. Managing Chronic Conditions: If you have any chronic medical conditions such as diabetes, hypertension, or thyroid disorders, work with your healthcare provider to ensure they are well-managed before conception. Proper management can significantly improve pregnancy outcomes.

Mental and Emotional Health

1. Stress Management: High levels of stress can affect fertility and overall well-being. Implement stress-reducing techniques such as mindfulness meditation, deep breathing exercises, and progressive muscle relaxation. Finding a healthy work-life balance and engaging in hobbies can also help manage stress.

2. Mental Health Support: Address any mental health concerns, such as anxiety or depression, before trying to conceive. Speak with a mental health professional for guidance and support. Therapy, counseling, and, if necessary, medication can be part of a comprehensive mental health plan.

3. Support Systems: Building a strong support network is essential. Surround yourself with family, friends, and a supportive partner who can provide emotional and practical support throughout your journey to parenthood. Joining support groups or online communities can also offer valuable connections and shared experiences.

Lifestyle and Environmental Factors

1. Environmental Exposures: Be aware of potential environmental hazards that could affect fertility and pregnancy. Limit exposure to harmful chemicals, pesticides, and pollutants. Opt for natural cleaning products, avoid excessive use of plastics, and be cautious with personal care products.

2. Occupational Hazards: If your job involves exposure to harmful substances or high levels of stress, discuss potential risks with your employer and healthcare provider. They may recommend adjustments or protective measures to ensure a safe working environment.

3. Vaccinations: Ensure you are up-to-date on all recommended vaccinations before conception. Vaccines protect against infections that could harm you or your developing baby. Common pre-pregnancy vaccines include MMR (measles, mumps, rubella), varicella (chickenpox), and the influenza vaccine.

4. Preconception Counseling: Consider attending preconception counseling sessions with your partner. These sessions provide an opportunity to discuss your plans, address any concerns, and receive comprehensive guidance from a healthcare professional.

Ensuring Wellness During Pregnancy

Once you conceive, maintaining wellness throughout pregnancy is crucial for the health of both mother and baby. This section will cover essential aspects of prenatal care, nutrition, exercise, mental health, and lifestyle adjustments to ensure a healthy pregnancy.

Prenatal Care

1. Regular Prenatal Visits: Schedule your first prenatal visit as soon as you confirm your pregnancy. Regular checkups with your healthcare provider are essential for monitoring your health and the development of your baby. These visits typically include:

- **Physical Examinations:** Assessing your overall health, weight gain, blood pressure, and fetal growth.
- **Ultrasounds:** Monitoring fetal development and detecting any potential issues.
- **Blood Tests:** Checking for anemia, gestational diabetes, and other conditions.
- **Urine Tests:** Screening for infections and protein levels.

2. Prenatal Vitamins: Continue taking prenatal vitamins throughout your pregnancy. These supplements provide essential nutrients such as folic acid, iron, calcium, and DHA (an omega-3 fatty acid). Follow your healthcare provider's recommendations for dosage and specific supplements.

3. Managing Common Pregnancy Symptoms: Pregnancy can bring various physical changes and symptoms. Some common issues and their management include:

- **Morning Sickness:** Eat small, frequent meals, stay hydrated, and avoid triggers. Ginger and vitamin B6 supplements may help.

- **Fatigue:** Prioritize rest, maintain a balanced diet, and engage in light exercise to boost energy levels.
- **Heartburn:** Eat smaller meals, avoid spicy and fatty foods, and elevate your head while sleeping.
- **Back Pain:** Practice good posture, use supportive pillows, and engage in gentle exercises like prenatal yoga.

Nutrition During Pregnancy

1. Balanced Diet: A nutritious diet is vital for the health of both mother and baby. Focus on a variety of foods to ensure you receive all necessary nutrients:

- **Protein:** Essential for fetal growth. Include lean meats, fish, eggs, beans, and nuts.
- **Calcium:** Supports bone development. Consume dairy products, fortified plant milks, and leafy greens.
- **Iron:** Prevents anemia. Include red meat, poultry, fish, beans, and fortified cereals.
- **Folic Acid:** Prevents neural tube defects. Continue taking a supplement and eat folate-rich foods like leafy greens and citrus fruits.
- **Fiber:** Prevents constipation. Include whole grains, fruits, vegetables, and legumes.

2. Hydration: Stay well-hydrated by drinking plenty of water throughout the day. Proper hydration supports blood volume expansion and helps prevent constipation.

3. Foods to Avoid: Certain foods can pose risks during pregnancy. Avoid:

- **Raw or Undercooked Seafood and Meat:** To prevent foodborne illnesses.
- **Unpasteurized Dairy Products and Juices:** To avoid harmful bacteria.
- **Certain Fish High in Mercury:** Such as shark, swordfish, king mackerel, and tilefish. Opt for low-mercury fish like salmon and shrimp.
- **Caffeine:** Limit intake to 200 milligrams per day (about one 12-ounce cup of coffee).

Exercise During Pregnancy

1. Benefits of Exercise: Regular physical activity during pregnancy offers numerous benefits, including improved mood, better sleep, reduced risk of gestational diabetes, and easier labor and delivery. Aim for at least 150 minutes of moderate-intensity exercise per week.

2. Safe Exercises: Choose activities that are safe and comfortable for you:

- **Walking:** A low-impact exercise that can be done throughout pregnancy.
- **Swimming:** Provides a full-body workout without putting stress on your joints.
- **Prenatal Yoga:** Improves flexibility, strength, and relaxation.
- **Pelvic Floor Exercises:** Strengthens the muscles that support the bladder, uterus, and bowels.

3. Exercises to Avoid: Certain activities should be avoided during pregnancy:

- **Contact Sports:** Such as soccer, basketball, and martial arts.
- **High-Impact Activities:** Like running or jumping, especially in the later stages of pregnancy.
- **Hot Yoga or Hot Pilates:** To avoid overheating.

Mental and Emotional Health During Pregnancy

1. Emotional Well-being: Pregnancy can bring a range of emotions, from joy to anxiety. It's important to take care of your mental health. Practice self-care by engaging in activities that bring you joy and relaxation.

Spend time with loved ones, pursue hobbies, and prioritize rest.

2. Support Systems: Surround yourself with a strong support network of family, friends, and your partner. Open communication with your support system can help you navigate the emotional ups and downs of pregnancy.

3. Professional Help: If you experience persistent feelings of sadness, anxiety, or depression, seek help from a mental health professional. Therapy or counseling can provide valuable support and coping strategies.

Lifestyle Adjustments

1. Avoiding Harmful Substances: Continue to avoid tobacco, alcohol, and recreational drugs during pregnancy. These substances can harm your baby and increase the risk of complications.

2. Safe Medications: Consult your healthcare provider before taking any medications, including over-the-counter drugs and supplements. Some medications may not be safe during pregnancy.

3. Environmental Safety: Minimize exposure to environmental hazards. Avoid harsh chemicals, opt for natural cleaning products, and reduce exposure to pollutants.

4. Travel Considerations: If you plan to travel during pregnancy, consult your healthcare provider for advice. Travel during the second trimester is generally considered safest. When flying, stay hydrated, move around frequently, and wear compression stockings to reduce the risk of blood clots.

Preparing for Childbirth

1. Childbirth Education Classes: Enroll in childbirth education classes to learn about the labor and delivery process, pain management options, and postpartum care. These classes can help you feel more prepared and confident.

2. Birth Plan: Create a birth plan outlining your preferences for labor and delivery. Include details such as pain relief options, who you want present, and any special requests. Share your plan with your healthcare provider and birthing team.

3. Packing for the Hospital: Prepare a hospital bag with essentials for you, your partner, and your baby. Include items such as comfortable clothing, toiletries, baby clothes, and important documents.

4. Postpartum Support: Plan for the postpartum period by arranging for support. This may include help with household tasks, meals, and childcare. Discuss your postpartum care plan with your healthcare provider to ensure you have the resources you need.

Ensuring wellness during pregnancy involves a comprehensive approach that includes regular prenatal care, a balanced diet, safe exercise, mental health support, and lifestyle adjustments. By taking these steps, you can promote the health and well-being of both yourself and your baby, setting the stage for a healthy pregnancy and childbirth experience.

Chapter 5: Early Years: Birth to Toddlerhood

Developmental Milestones and Health Monitoring

The early years of a child's life, from birth to toddlerhood, are a period of rapid growth and development. During this time, your child will achieve numerous developmental milestones, which are critical indicators of their physical, cognitive, and emotional progress. Understanding these milestones and monitoring your child's health are essential components of ensuring their overall well-being.

Physical Development

From the moment of birth, infants begin a remarkable journey of physical growth. The first year of life is characterized by significant changes, including doubling or even tripling their birth weight, growing in length, and developing motor skills. These milestones are crucial markers of healthy development.

0-3 Months:

- **Motor Skills:** Newborns exhibit reflexive movements, such as the rooting and sucking reflexes. By three months, they can lift their heads while lying on their stomachs and start to gain control over their hand movements.

- **Sensory Development:** Infants begin to focus their eyes, follow moving objects, and recognize familiar faces and voices. They start responding to sounds by turning their heads towards the source.

4-6 Months:

- **Motor Skills:** By this age, infants can roll over, sit with support, and bring objects to their mouths. They begin to reach and grasp for toys, developing hand-eye coordination.
- **Social Development:** Babies start to smile, laugh, and show more interest in their surroundings. They may recognize their parents and caregivers and respond to affection.

7-12 Months:

- **Motor Skills:** This period is marked by significant mobility. Babies learn to sit without support, crawl, stand with assistance, and eventually take their first steps. Fine motor skills improve as they pick up small objects using their thumb and forefinger.

- **Cognitive Development:** Infants start to understand simple words and commands. They enjoy playing peek-a-boo, exploring their environment, and imitating sounds and gestures.

1-2 Years:

- **Motor Skills:** Toddlers become more independent and adventurous. They can walk, run, climb stairs, and throw a ball. Fine motor skills continue to develop, allowing them to stack blocks, scribble with crayons, and feed themselves with utensils.
- **Language Development:** Vocabulary expands rapidly during this stage. Toddlers begin to use simple sentences, name familiar objects, and follow basic instructions. They also start to engage in pretend play and express a range of emotions.

Cognitive and Emotional Development

Cognitive and emotional development are intertwined and play a significant role in a child's early years. Cognitive development refers to the growth of thinking, reasoning, and problem-solving abilities, while emotional development involves understanding and managing emotions, forming relationships, and developing self-awareness.

0-3 Months:

- **Cognitive Development:** Infants are naturally curious and begin to explore their environment through their senses. They start to recognize patterns, such as the routine of feeding and sleeping.
- **Emotional Development:** Newborns express their needs through crying and begin to form attachments to their caregivers. They find comfort in familiar voices and touch.

4-6 Months:

- **Cognitive Development:** Babies become more aware of cause-and-effect relationships. They enjoy shaking rattles, dropping toys, and observing the results of their actions.
- **Emotional Development:** Infants show a broader range of emotions, including joy, frustration, and curiosity. They may develop separation anxiety when away from their primary caregivers.

7-12 Months:

- **Cognitive Development:** Babies engage in more complex exploration, such as opening and closing objects, stacking blocks, and searching for hidden items. They begin to understand object permanence—the concept that objects continue to exist even when out of sight.
- **Emotional Development:** Infants start to form attachments to specific people and may show preferences for certain toys or activities. They enjoy social interactions, such as clapping hands and playing simple games.

1-2 Years:

- **Cognitive Development:** Toddlers demonstrate problem-solving skills by figuring out how to open doors, fit shapes into corresponding holes, and complete simple puzzles. They begin to understand symbolic play, using objects to represent other things.
- **Emotional Development:** Toddlers experience a wide range of emotions and begin to assert their independence. They may have temper tantrums as they navigate frustration and learn to

communicate their needs. They also develop empathy and start to show concern for others.

Health Monitoring

Regular health monitoring is essential during the early years to ensure that your child is growing and developing as expected. Pediatricians and healthcare providers play a crucial role in this process, conducting routine check-ups, administering vaccinations, and providing guidance on nutrition, safety, and overall well-being.

Well-Baby Visits: Well-baby visits are scheduled check-ups that occur frequently during the first year and then periodically throughout early childhood. These visits are opportunities to monitor your child's growth, discuss any concerns, and receive vaccinations.

- **Newborn Visit:** Typically within the first week after birth, this visit includes a thorough examination, weight check, and discussion of feeding and sleep patterns.
- **1-2 Months:** Monitoring growth, head circumference, and developmental milestones. Discussion of breastfeeding or formula feeding and introduction of immunizations.

- **4-6 Months:** Continued assessment of growth and development, including motor skills and sensory responses. Introduction of solid foods and age-appropriate feeding advice.
- **9-12 Months:** Evaluation of mobility, language development, and social interactions. Discussion of safety measures as your child becomes more mobile.
- **15-18 Months:** Assessment of cognitive and emotional development, including language skills and social behaviors. Continued immunizations and guidance on nutrition and sleep.
- **2 Years:** Comprehensive evaluation of physical, cognitive, and emotional milestones. Discussion of toilet training, nutrition, and early childhood education.

Growth Charts: Pediatricians use growth charts to track your child's height, weight, and head circumference over time. These charts help identify patterns of growth and ensure that your child is developing within a healthy range. If any concerns arise, your healthcare provider may recommend further evaluation or interventions.

Developmental Screenings: Developmental screenings are tools used to assess your child's progress in areas such as motor skills, language, social interactions, and problem-solving. These screenings help identify any delays or concerns early on, allowing for timely intervention and support.

Hearing and Vision Screenings: Hearing and vision are critical for overall development. Early detection of hearing or vision issues can prevent potential delays in language and cognitive skills. Pediatricians may conduct screenings or refer you to specialists if needed.

Vaccine Decisions for Infants and Toddlers

Vaccination is one of the most effective ways to protect your child from serious and potentially life-threatening diseases. During infancy and toddlerhood, children receive several important vaccines that help build immunity and prevent the spread of infectious diseases.

The Importance of Vaccination

Vaccines work by stimulating the immune system to recognize and fight specific pathogens, such as viruses or bacteria, without causing the disease itself. This process involves introducing a harmless component of the pathogen, such as a protein or a weakened form, which trains the immune system to respond effectively if exposed to the actual disease in the future.

The benefits of vaccination are numerous:

- **Disease Prevention:** Vaccines protect against diseases such as measles, mumps, rubella, polio, diphtheria, pertussis (whooping cough), and more. These diseases can cause severe complications and even death, especially in young children.
- **Community Immunity:** When a significant portion of the population is vaccinated, it creates herd immunity, reducing the spread of diseases and protecting those who cannot be vaccinated due to medical reasons.
- **Long-Term Health:** Vaccines help prevent chronic health conditions that can result from infections. For example, the hepatitis B vaccine prevents liver disease and cancer caused by the hepatitis B virus.

Recommended Vaccination Schedule

The Centers for Disease Control and Prevention (CDC) and other health organizations provide recommended vaccination schedules to ensure that children receive vaccines at the appropriate times for maximum protection. Below is an overview of the recommended vaccines for infants and toddlers:

Birth:

- **Hepatitis B (HepB):** The first dose is given at birth to protect against hepatitis B, a virus that can cause chronic liver disease.

2 Months:

- **Diphtheria, Tetanus, and Acellular Pertussis (DTaP):** Protects against diphtheria, tetanus, and pertussis.
- **Haemophilus Influenzae Type B (Hib):** Protects against infections caused by Haemophilus influenzae type b, such as meningitis and pneumonia.
- **Inactivated Poliovirus (IPV):** Protects against polio, a virus that can cause paralysis.
- **Pneumococcal Conjugate (PCV13):** Protects against pneumococcal infections, which can cause pneumonia, meningitis, and sepsis.
- **Rotavirus (RV):** Protects against rotavirus, a virus that causes severe diarrhea and dehydration.

4 Months:

- **DTaP:** Second dose.
- **Hib:** Second dose.

- **IPV:** Second dose.
- **PCV13:** Second dose.
- **RV:** Second dose.

6 Months:

- **DTaP:** Third dose.
- **Hib:** Third dose (if needed).
- **IPV:** Third dose.
- **PCV13:** Third dose.
- **RV:** Third dose (if needed).
- **Influenza (Flu):** Annual vaccination begins at 6 months to protect against the flu.

12-15 Months:

- **Hib:** Final dose.
- **PCV13:** Final dose.
- **Measles, Mumps, and Rubella (MMR):** Protects against measles, mumps, and rubella.
- **Varicella (Chickenpox):** Protects against chickenpox.
- **Hepatitis A (HepA):** First dose to protect against hepatitis A, a virus that causes liver disease.

15-18 Months:

- **DTaP:** Fourth dose.

18-24 Months:

- **HepA:** Second dose (6 months after the first dose).

It is important to follow the recommended vaccination schedule to ensure that your child receives the necessary protection at the appropriate times. Delaying or skipping vaccines can leave your child vulnerable to diseases that are preventable through vaccination.

Addressing Vaccine Concerns

As a parent, it is natural to have questions and concerns about vaccines. Addressing these concerns with accurate information and evidence-based answers can help you make informed decisions for your child's health.

Safety and Side Effects:

- **Common Side Effects:** Vaccines are generally safe, but like any medical intervention, they can have side effects. Common side effects include mild fever, redness or swelling at the injection site, and fussiness. These side effects are usually short-lived and indicate that the body is building immunity.

- **Serious Side Effects:** Serious side effects are rare. The benefits of vaccination far outweigh the risks. Monitoring systems, such as the Vaccine Adverse Event Reporting System (VAERS), help track and investigate any adverse events.

Vaccine Ingredients:

- **Understanding Ingredients:** Vaccines contain antigens (components that stimulate the immune response), preservatives, stabilizers, and adjuvants (substances that enhance the immune response). Each ingredient serves a specific purpose in ensuring the vaccine's safety and efficacy.
- **Thimerosal:** Concerns about thimerosal, a mercury-containing preservative, have been addressed. Thimerosal is no longer used in most childhood vaccines, and extensive research has shown no link between thimerosal and autism.

Autism and Vaccines:

- **Debunking Myths:** The claim that vaccines cause autism has been thoroughly debunked by numerous studies. The original study that suggested a link was found to be fraudulent and was retracted. Major health organizations, including the CDC, the World Health Organization (WHO), and the American Academy of Pediatrics (AAP), confirm that vaccines do not cause autism.

Alternative Vaccination Schedules:

- **Evaluating Alternatives:** Some parents consider alternative vaccination schedules. It is important to discuss these options with your healthcare provider. Delaying vaccines can leave your child unprotected against preventable diseases during critical periods.

- **Evidence-Based Decisions:** Sticking to the recommended vaccination schedule ensures that your child receives protection when it is most needed. Deviating from the schedule can increase the risk of outbreaks and reduce the effectiveness of herd immunity.

Practical Tips for Vaccine-Friendly Parenting

Being a vaccine-friendly parent involves practical steps and strategies to ensure your child's health and well-being:

1. **Educate Yourself:** Take the time to learn about vaccines, how they work, and the diseases they prevent. Use reputable sources such as healthcare providers, scientific journals, and trusted health organizations.

2. **Communicate with Your Healthcare Provider:** Establish a trusting relationship with your child's healthcare provider. Ask questions, express concerns, and seek their guidance in making vaccination decisions.

3. **Stay Informed:** Keep up-to-date with the latest information on vaccines and vaccination schedules. Health recommendations can evolve, and staying informed ensures you are making decisions based on current evidence.

4. **Respect Others' Decisions:** Understand that every parent wants the best for their child. Respect the decisions of others, even if they differ from your own, and engage in respectful conversations about vaccines.

5. **Create a Supportive Environment:** Foster a positive environment where your child feels safe and supported during vaccinations. Comfort them

with soothing words, hugs, and rewards for their bravery.

The early years of your child's life are a time of rapid growth, development, and important health decisions. By understanding developmental milestones, monitoring your child's health, and making informed vaccine decisions, you are laying the foundation for their long-term well-being. Vaccination is a powerful tool in protecting your child from serious diseases and contributing to the health of your community. Embrace a vaccine-friendly approach to parenting, grounded in knowledge, trust, and a commitment to your child's health.

Chapter 6: Childhood: Preschool and School-Age Years

Well-Child Visits and Developmental Assessments

Well-child visits are a fundamental component of pediatric healthcare, playing a crucial role in monitoring and promoting the health and development of children from infancy through adolescence. These visits provide an opportunity for healthcare providers to assess a child's growth, development, and overall well-being, as well as to offer guidance to parents on a range of topics, from nutrition to behavior.

Importance of Well-Child Visits

Well-child visits are scheduled regularly throughout a child's life, typically more frequently during the early years and then annually during the school-age years. These visits are designed to:

1. **Monitor Growth and Development**: Healthcare providers track a child's physical growth (height, weight, and head circumference) and developmental milestones (such as speech, motor skills, and social interactions). These assessments

help identify any potential delays or concerns early, allowing for timely intervention.

2. **Provide Preventive Care**: Immunizations, vision and hearing screenings, and other preventive measures are an integral part of well-child visits. Vaccinations protect children from serious infectious diseases, while screenings help detect issues that may affect learning and development.

3. **Offer Parental Guidance**: Pediatricians provide parents with valuable advice on nutrition, sleep, safety, discipline, and other aspects of child-rearing. This guidance is tailored to the child's age and developmental stage, helping parents navigate the challenges of raising healthy children.

4. **Build a Healthcare Relationship**: Regular visits help establish a trusting relationship between the family and the healthcare provider. This relationship is important for addressing health concerns, ensuring continuity of care, and supporting the overall health of the child.

Components of Well-Child Visits

Each well-child visit is tailored to the child's age and developmental stage. Key components typically include:

1. **Physical Examination**: The healthcare provider conducts a thorough physical examination to assess the child's overall health. This includes checking vital signs, examining the eyes, ears, nose, throat, heart, lungs, abdomen, skin, and musculoskeletal system.

2. **Growth Measurements**: The child's height, weight, and head circumference (for younger children) are measured and plotted on growth charts. These charts help track growth patterns and identify any deviations from the expected range.

3. **Developmental Screening**: Developmental assessments evaluate the child's progress in areas such as language, motor skills, cognitive abilities, and social interactions. Standardized tools and questionnaires may be used to screen for developmental delays or concerns.

4. **Immunizations**: Vaccinations are administered according to the recommended schedule to protect against diseases such as measles, mumps, rubella, polio, and influenza. The healthcare provider also discusses the benefits and potential side effects of each vaccine with the parents.

5. **Vision and Hearing Screenings**: Regular screenings help detect vision and hearing

problems that could affect learning and development. Early identification and intervention are crucial for addressing these issues.

6. **Behavioral and Emotional Health**: The healthcare provider assesses the child's behavioral and emotional well-being, addressing any concerns related to anxiety, depression, attention, or behavior. This assessment is especially important during the school-age years when children may face new social and academic challenges.

7. **Parental Education and Guidance**: The pediatrician provides parents with information on a range of topics, including nutrition, sleep, physical activity, safety, and discipline. This guidance is tailored to the child's age and developmental stage, helping parents support their child's growth and development.

8. **Addressing Parental Concerns**: Parents are encouraged to share any concerns or questions they may have about their child's health, development, or behavior. The healthcare provider offers advice and support, helping parents navigate common challenges and make informed decisions.

Developmental Assessments

Developmental assessments are a key component of well-child visits, providing valuable insights into a child's progress in various domains. These assessments help identify potential developmental delays or concerns early, allowing for timely intervention and support.

Domains of Development

1. **Cognitive Development**: Cognitive development refers to the child's ability to think, learn, and solve problems. During preschool and school-age years, children develop important cognitive skills such as memory, attention, and reasoning. Developmental assessments evaluate these skills through age-appropriate tasks and activities.

2. **Language Development**: Language development includes both receptive language (understanding) and expressive language (speaking). Children's language skills progress rapidly during the preschool years, and continued development is essential for academic success. Assessments may involve evaluating vocabulary, sentence structure, and communication abilities.

3. **Motor Development**: Motor development encompasses both fine motor skills (such as writing and drawing) and gross motor skills (such as running and jumping). Assessments evaluate the child's coordination, strength, and dexterity, helping identify any delays or difficulties that may require intervention.

4. **Social and Emotional Development**: Social and emotional development involves the child's ability to form relationships, manage emotions, and navigate social interactions. Assessments may explore the child's ability to cooperate, share, empathize, and regulate emotions. These skills are crucial for building positive relationships and succeeding in school.

5. **Adaptive Development**: Adaptive development refers to the child's ability to perform everyday tasks and activities independently. This includes skills such as dressing, feeding, and using the bathroom. Assessments help identify any areas where the child may need additional support or intervention.

Common Developmental Assessments

1. **Ages and Stages Questionnaires (ASQ)**: The ASQ is a widely used screening tool that assesses

development across multiple domains. Parents complete questionnaires that evaluate their child's skills and behaviors, providing a comprehensive overview of development.

2. **Denver Developmental Screening Test (DDST)**: The DDST assesses children's development in four domains: personal-social, fine motor-adaptive, language, and gross motor. It involves direct observation and parent interviews to evaluate developmental milestones.

3. **Bayley Scales of Infant and Toddler Development**: This comprehensive assessment evaluates cognitive, language, motor, social-emotional, and adaptive development in young children. It provides detailed information on a child's strengths and areas of concern.

4. **Battelle Developmental Inventory (BDI)**: The BDI assesses development across five domains: personal-social, adaptive, motor, communication, and cognitive. It is used to identify developmental delays and plan interventions.

5. **Pediatric Evaluation of Disability Inventory (PEDI)**: The PEDI assesses functional abilities and performance in daily activities, providing information on a child's self-care, mobility, and social function.

Early Intervention and Support

Early identification of developmental delays or concerns is crucial for providing timely intervention and support. Well-child visits and developmental assessments help identify children who may benefit from early intervention services, such as speech therapy, occupational therapy, or specialized educational programs. Early intervention can significantly improve outcomes for children with developmental delays, helping them reach their full potential.

Managing Common Childhood Illnesses

Preschool and school-age children are often exposed to a variety of illnesses as they interact with peers and explore their environment. Managing these common childhood illnesses effectively is essential for maintaining their health and well-being.

Common Childhood Illnesses

1. **Colds and Upper Respiratory Infections**: Colds are caused by viruses and are characterized by symptoms such as runny nose, cough, sore throat,

and fever. These infections are common among young children and typically resolve on their own with supportive care.

2. **Ear Infections**: Ear infections, or otitis media, occur when fluid builds up in the middle ear and becomes infected. Symptoms include ear pain, fever, and irritability. Treatment may involve pain relief and, in some cases, antibiotics.

3. **Gastroenteritis**: Gastroenteritis, also known as stomach flu, is an infection of the digestive system that causes diarrhea, vomiting, and abdominal pain. It is usually caused by viruses and can lead to dehydration if not managed properly.

4. **Hand, Foot, and Mouth Disease**: This viral illness is characterized by fever, sores in the mouth, and a rash on the hands and feet. It is common in young children and usually resolves on its own with supportive care.

5. **Conjunctivitis (Pink Eye)**: Conjunctivitis is an infection or inflammation of the conjunctiva, the thin membrane that lines the eye. It can be caused by viruses, bacteria, or allergens and is characterized by redness, itching, and discharge.

6. **Croup**: Croup is a viral infection that causes inflammation of the upper airway, leading to a distinctive barking cough and difficulty breathing.

It is common in young children and can often be managed with supportive care.

7. **Asthma**: Asthma is a chronic condition characterized by inflammation and narrowing of the airways, leading to wheezing, coughing, and shortness of breath. Managing asthma involves avoiding triggers, using medications, and developing an asthma action plan.

8. **Allergies**: Allergies occur when the immune system overreacts to substances such as pollen, dust mites, or certain foods. Symptoms can include sneezing, itching, and skin rashes. Management involves avoiding allergens and using medications as needed.

Management and Care

1. **Symptomatic Relief**: Many common childhood illnesses are viral and do not require antibiotics. Symptomatic relief includes measures such as providing fluids, ensuring rest, and using over-the-counter medications to reduce fever and alleviate pain.

2. **Hydration**: Keeping children hydrated is essential, especially during illnesses that cause vomiting or diarrhea. Oral rehydration solutions

can help prevent dehydration by replacing lost fluids and electrolytes.

3. **Monitoring Symptoms**: Parents should monitor their child's symptoms and seek medical advice if there are signs of worsening illness, such as high fever, difficulty breathing, persistent vomiting, or severe pain.

4. **Infection Control**: Preventing the spread of infections involves practicing good hygiene, such as regular handwashing, covering the mouth and nose when coughing or sneezing, and keeping sick children home from school or daycare.

5. **Medication Management**: When medications are prescribed, it is important to follow the dosage instructions carefully and complete the full course of treatment. Overuse or misuse of antibiotics can lead to antibiotic resistance and other complications.

6. **Home Care and Comfort**: Providing comfort and reassurance to a sick child is an important aspect of care. This includes creating a calm and soothing environment, offering favorite foods and drinks, and using comfort measures such as warm baths or humidifiers.

When to Seek Medical Attention

While many common childhood illnesses can be managed at home, there are situations where medical attention is necessary. Parents should seek medical advice if their child experiences:

- High fever (above 102°F or 39°C) that persists for more than a few days
- Difficulty breathing or rapid breathing
- Severe or persistent pain, especially in the ear or abdomen
- Signs of dehydration, such as dry mouth, sunken eyes, or reduced urine output
- Persistent vomiting or diarrhea
- Rash that spreads or looks infected
- Lethargy or unusual drowsiness
- Seizures or convulsions
- Symptoms that worsen or do not improve with home care

Preventive Measures

Preventing illness is an important aspect of maintaining children's health. Key preventive measures include:

1. **Vaccination**: Ensuring that children are up-to-date with their vaccinations helps protect them from serious infectious diseases. Vaccines are one

of the most effective tools in preventing illness and maintaining public health.

2. **Healthy Lifestyle**: Encouraging a healthy lifestyle with a balanced diet, regular physical activity, and adequate sleep supports the immune system and overall well-being.

3. **Hygiene Practices**: Teaching children good hygiene practices, such as handwashing, covering their mouth and nose when coughing or sneezing, and avoiding sharing utensils, helps prevent the spread of infections.

4. **Avoiding Sick Contacts**: Limiting exposure to individuals who are sick can help reduce the risk of illness. This is especially important during outbreaks of contagious diseases.

5. **Regular Check-Ups**: Regular well-child visits allow healthcare providers to monitor children's health, provide preventive care, and address any concerns early.

The preschool and school-age years are a critical period for growth and development. Well-child visits and developmental assessments play a vital role in monitoring children's health and ensuring they are on track to reach their full potential. By managing common childhood illnesses effectively and taking preventive measures, parents can support their children's well-being and help them thrive.

This chapter has provided an overview of the importance of well-child visits, the components of these visits, and the role of developmental assessments in identifying and addressing potential concerns.

It has also covered the management of common childhood illnesses, including symptoms, treatment, and preventive measures. By being informed and proactive, parents can navigate the challenges of childhood health and support their children's healthy development.

Chapter 7: Adolescence: Preparing for Young Adulthood

Health and Wellness in Teenage Years

Adolescence is a critical period of growth and development, marked by significant physical, emotional, and social changes. It is a time when children transition into young adulthood, taking on more responsibility for their own health and wellness. As a parent, guiding your adolescent through these years requires a balanced approach that supports their independence while ensuring they make informed and healthy choices.

During adolescence, the body undergoes rapid changes. Puberty brings about physical growth, hormonal shifts, and sexual maturation. These changes can be challenging and sometimes overwhelming for teenagers, making it essential for parents to provide support and education. Understanding the basics of adolescent development can help you better support your child during this transformative period.

Physical Development

The physical changes that occur during adolescence are perhaps the most noticeable. These include growth spurts, the development of secondary sexual characteristics, and changes in body composition. Boys and girls experience these changes at different rates, but both will go through similar stages of development.

Boys typically experience a growth spurt between the ages of 12 and 16, gaining height and muscle mass. Their voices deepen, and facial and body hair begins to grow. Girls usually start their growth spurt earlier, around ages 10 to 14, and develop breast tissue, wider hips, and menstruation.

These physical changes can affect teenagers' self-esteem and body image. It's important to foster a positive body image by encouraging healthy eating, regular physical activity, and self-acceptance. Adolescents should be reminded that everyone develops at their own pace and that comparing themselves to others is not productive.

Emotional and Social Development

Emotional and social development is equally significant during adolescence. Teenagers start to form their own identities, separate from their parents, and place greater importance on peer relationships. They may experience mood swings, increased sensitivity, and a desire for independence.

As a parent, maintaining open communication is crucial. Encourage your adolescent to express their feelings and listen without judgment. This can help them navigate the emotional ups and downs of adolescence and develop healthy coping mechanisms.

Peer pressure becomes more influential during these years. Adolescents may feel pressured to conform to their peers' behaviors, which can sometimes lead to risky activities such as experimenting with drugs or alcohol. Educating your teenager about the potential consequences of these behaviors and promoting positive peer relationships can mitigate these risks.

Mental Health

Mental health is a critical aspect of adolescent wellness. Teenagers may face various stressors, including academic pressures, social challenges, and family dynamics. These stressors can contribute to mental health issues such as anxiety, depression, and eating disorders.

Promoting mental health involves creating a supportive environment where your adolescent feels safe and valued. Encourage healthy habits such as regular exercise, balanced nutrition, and sufficient sleep. Be vigilant for signs of mental health problems, such as changes in behavior, withdrawal from activities, or a decline in academic performance. If you suspect your teenager is struggling, seek professional help promptly.

Nutrition and Physical Activity

Proper nutrition and regular physical activity are essential for the health and development of adolescents. A balanced diet that includes a variety of fruits, vegetables, whole grains, lean proteins, and healthy fats provides the necessary nutrients for growth and energy.

Teenagers often have busy schedules, which can make healthy eating challenging. Encourage your adolescent to make nutritious food choices and limit the consumption of sugary snacks and beverages. Family meals can be an excellent opportunity to model healthy eating habits and spend quality time together.

Physical activity is equally important. Encourage your adolescent to engage in regular exercise, whether through sports, dance, or other activities they enjoy. Exercise not only supports physical health but also benefits mental well-being by reducing stress and improving mood.

Sleep

Sleep is often overlooked, but it is vital for adolescent health. Teenagers need more sleep than adults, typically around 8-10 hours per night. However, many adolescents do not get enough sleep due to busy schedules, electronic device use, and social activities.

Lack of sleep can affect mood, cognitive function, and overall health. Encourage your teenager to establish a regular sleep routine, limit screen time before bed, and create a conducive sleep environment. Adequate sleep is essential for academic performance, emotional regulation, and physical health.

Vaccination Considerations for Adolescents

Vaccination remains a crucial component of adolescent health. As children grow into teenagers, they may need additional vaccines to protect against diseases that become more relevant during these years. Understanding the recommended vaccines and their importance can help you ensure your adolescent is well-protected.

Tetanus, Diphtheria, and Pertussis (Tdap) Vaccine

The Tdap vaccine is essential for adolescents, as it provides protection against tetanus, diphtheria, and pertussis (whooping cough). The Tdap booster is typically recommended around the age of 11 or 12. Pertussis, in particular, is highly contagious and can cause severe illness, especially in infants and young children. By vaccinating adolescents, we help prevent the spread of these diseases within the community.

Human Papillomavirus (HPV) Vaccine

The HPV vaccine protects against the human papillomavirus, which can lead to various cancers, including cervical, anal, and throat cancers. The vaccine is most effective when administered before exposure to the virus, which is why it is recommended for preteens aged 11 to 12. However, it can be given as early as age 9 and up to age 26 for those who did not receive it earlier.

HPV vaccination is a critical preventive measure. Educating your adolescent about the benefits of the vaccine and addressing any concerns they may have can encourage vaccination compliance.

Meningococcal Vaccines

Meningococcal disease is a severe bacterial infection that can cause meningitis and bloodstream infections. Adolescents are at increased risk, especially those living in close quarters, such as college dormitories. Two types of meningococcal vaccines are recommended for adolescents:

1. **Meningococcal conjugate vaccine (MenACWY)**: This vaccine protects against serogroups A, C, W, and Y. It is typically given at age 11 or 12, with a booster dose at age 16.
2. **Serogroup B meningococcal vaccine (MenB)**: This vaccine protects against serogroup B. It is recommended for adolescents aged 16 to 23, depending on individual risk factors.

Ensuring your adolescent receives these vaccines can prevent life-threatening infections and their complications.

Influenza Vaccine

The annual influenza vaccine is recommended for all individuals aged 6 months and older, including adolescents. Influenza can cause severe illness and complications, particularly in vulnerable populations. Vaccinating your adolescent against the flu not only protects them but also helps reduce the spread of the virus in the community.

Hepatitis A and B Vaccines

Hepatitis A and B are viral infections that affect the liver. The hepatitis B vaccine is usually given during infancy, but some adolescents may need catch-up doses if they were not vaccinated earlier. The hepatitis A vaccine is recommended for all children aged 1 year and older, and adolescents who have not previously received it should also be vaccinated.

Varicella (Chickenpox) Vaccine

The varicella vaccine protects against chickenpox, a highly contagious disease that can cause severe complications. Adolescents who have not previously been vaccinated or who have not had chickenpox should receive two doses of the vaccine.

Measles, Mumps, and Rubella (MMR) Vaccine

The MMR vaccine is typically given during early childhood, but some adolescents may need catch-up doses if they were not vaccinated earlier. Measles, mumps, and rubella are serious diseases that can cause significant health problems. Ensuring your adolescent is up-to-date on the MMR vaccine is crucial for their health and for public health.

Polio Vaccine

The polio vaccine is usually administered during childhood, but adolescents who did not complete the series should receive catch-up doses. Polio is a crippling and potentially deadly disease, and vaccination is essential to prevent its resurgence.

Importance of Keeping Vaccination Records

Maintaining accurate vaccination records is essential for ensuring your adolescent is up-to-date with their immunizations. Keep a record of all vaccines received, including the dates and any adverse reactions. This information can be valuable for school entry, travel, and healthcare purposes.

If your adolescent is unsure about their vaccination status, consult with your healthcare provider. They can review medical records and, if necessary, conduct blood tests to determine immunity levels.

Addressing Vaccine Hesitancy

Vaccine hesitancy can be a barrier to ensuring your adolescent is fully vaccinated. Concerns about vaccine safety, misinformation, and mistrust of the healthcare system can contribute to reluctance. Addressing these concerns with empathy and providing evidence-based information is crucial.

Engage in open and respectful conversations with your adolescent about the importance of vaccines. Encourage them to ask questions and express their concerns. Provide accurate information from trusted sources, such as healthcare providers and reputable health organizations.

It's also helpful to share personal stories and experiences. Hearing from peers, family members, or community leaders who support vaccination can positively influence your adolescent's views.

Promoting Vaccination in Schools and Communities

Schools and communities play a significant role in promoting vaccination. Many schools require proof of immunization for enrollment, which helps ensure a healthy learning environment. Support vaccination initiatives in schools and advocate for policies that protect public health.

Community engagement is also vital. Participate in local health campaigns, attend informational sessions, and collaborate with healthcare providers to raise awareness about the importance of vaccines. By fostering a culture of vaccination, you contribute to the overall health and well-being of your community.

Adolescence is a transformative period of growth and development. As your child transitions into young adulthood, ensuring their health and wellness becomes increasingly important. By understanding the unique challenges and opportunities of adolescence, you can support your teenager in making informed and healthy choices.

Vaccination remains a cornerstone of adolescent health. Ensuring your adolescent is up-to-date with recommended vaccines protects them from serious diseases and contributes to the health of the community. Addressing vaccine hesitancy with empathy and providing accurate information can help overcome barriers to vaccination.

Remember, you are not alone in this journey. Healthcare providers, educators, and community organizations are valuable partners in promoting adolescent health. By working together, we can support our adolescents in achieving their full potential and building a healthier future.

As you navigate the complexities of adolescence, keep the lines of communication open, provide support and guidance, and empower your teenager to take responsibility for their health. With the right information and resources, you can help them thrive during these formative years and beyond.

Chapter 8: Communicating with Healthcare Providers

Advocating for Your Child's Health Needs

Advocating for your child's health needs is an essential part of parenting, especially when it comes to interactions with healthcare providers. Advocacy involves understanding your child's needs, effectively communicating them to healthcare professionals, and ensuring that your child's best interests are prioritized. This chapter will guide you through the process of advocating for your child's health, providing practical advice on how to navigate the healthcare system and build a collaborative relationship with healthcare providers.

Understanding Your Child's Health Needs

The first step in advocating for your child's health is to understand their specific needs. This involves being observant and informed about your child's health and developmental milestones. Regularly tracking your child's growth, behavior, and any symptoms or changes in their health can provide valuable information that can be shared with healthcare providers. Here are some key aspects to consider:

- **Developmental Milestones**: Keep track of your child's physical, cognitive, and social development. Knowing what milestones to expect at different ages can help you identify any potential concerns early.

- **Medical History**: Maintain a detailed record of your child's medical history, including vaccinations, illnesses, surgeries, allergies, and any chronic conditions. This information is crucial for healthcare providers to make informed decisions.

- **Symptoms and Changes**: Pay attention to any changes in your child's health, such as unusual symptoms, changes in behavior, or developmental delays. Documenting these changes can help healthcare providers understand your child's health better.

Effective Communication Strategies

Effective communication with healthcare providers is essential for advocating for your child's health needs. Here are some strategies to help you communicate more effectively:

- **Prepare for Appointments**: Before each appointment, make a list of questions or concerns you want to discuss with the healthcare provider. Bring any relevant medical records or documentation to the appointment.

- **Be Clear and Concise**: When describing your child's symptoms or concerns, be clear and concise. Use specific examples and avoid vague descriptions. For instance, instead of saying "My child is not feeling well," provide details such as "My child has had a fever of 102°F for the past two days and has been complaining of a sore throat."
- **Ask Questions**: Don't hesitate to ask questions if you don't understand something or need more information. Healthcare providers are there to help, and asking questions can ensure you fully understand your child's health and treatment options.
- **Take Notes**: During the appointment, take notes on what the healthcare provider says. This can help you remember important information and instructions later.
- **Follow-Up**: If you have additional questions or concerns after the appointment, don't hesitate to follow up with the healthcare provider. Clear and ongoing communication is key to effective healthcare advocacy.

Building a Collaborative Relationship

Building a collaborative relationship with healthcare providers is crucial for effective advocacy. This involves mutual respect, trust, and a willingness to work together for your child's best interests. Here are some tips for fostering a positive relationship:

- **Respect Expertise**: Recognize and respect the expertise and knowledge of healthcare providers. They have extensive training and experience in diagnosing and treating health conditions.
- **Share Your Knowledge**: You are the expert on your child's unique needs and behaviors. Share your observations and insights with the healthcare provider to help them understand your child's health better.
- **Be Honest and Open**: Honesty is essential in healthcare. Be open about your child's symptoms, medical history, and any concerns you have. This allows healthcare providers to make accurate assessments and provide appropriate care.
- **Stay Informed**: Stay informed about your child's health condition and treatment options. This enables you to have meaningful discussions with

healthcare providers and make informed decisions.

- **Express Gratitude**: Acknowledge and express gratitude for the care and support provided by healthcare providers. Positive reinforcement can strengthen your relationship and encourage ongoing collaboration.

Navigating the Healthcare System

Navigating the healthcare system can be complex, but understanding how it works can help you advocate more effectively for your child's health. Here are some key aspects to consider:

- **Understanding Healthcare Providers**: Healthcare providers include pediatricians, family doctors, specialists, nurses, and other professionals. Each has a specific role in your child's care. Understanding these roles can help you know whom to approach for different health concerns.
- **Healthcare Settings**: Healthcare services can be provided in various settings, including clinics, hospitals, urgent care centers, and specialist offices. Knowing which setting is appropriate for

your child's needs can help you access the right care promptly.

- **Insurance and Costs**: Understanding your health insurance coverage and any out-of-pocket costs is essential. Familiarize yourself with your insurance plan's benefits, network providers, and coverage limitations. This can help you avoid unexpected expenses and ensure your child receives necessary care.

- **Patient Rights and Responsibilities**: Be aware of your rights and responsibilities as a patient or parent of a patient. This includes the right to informed consent, privacy, and access to medical records, as well as the responsibility to provide accurate information and follow treatment plans.

Overcoming Communication Barriers

Effective communication with healthcare providers can sometimes be challenging due to various barriers. Identifying and addressing these barriers can improve your ability to advocate for your child's health. Here are some common barriers and strategies to overcome them:

- **Language Barriers**: If there is a language barrier, consider using translation services or bringing a bilingual friend or family member to appointments. Many healthcare facilities offer interpreter services to assist with communication.

- **Health Literacy**: Health literacy refers to the ability to understand and use health information. If medical terminology or instructions are confusing, ask healthcare providers to explain in simpler terms or provide written materials.

- **Cultural Differences**: Cultural beliefs and practices can influence health decisions and communication. Be open about your cultural preferences and ask healthcare providers to consider these in your child's care.

- **Emotional Stress**: Healthcare visits can be stressful, especially when discussing serious health concerns. If you feel overwhelmed, take a moment to collect your thoughts, or consider bringing a support person to appointments for emotional support.

Empowering Your Child in Healthcare Decisions

As your child grows, it's important to involve them in their healthcare decisions to the extent appropriate for their age and development. Empowering your child in healthcare decisions can foster independence and a sense of responsibility for their own health. Here are some tips for involving your child:

- **Educate Your Child**: Teach your child about their health condition and the importance of treatments and preventive care. Use age-appropriate language and materials to help them understand.
- **Encourage Questions**: Encourage your child to ask questions during healthcare visits. This can help them feel more involved and less anxious about medical appointments.
- **Involve Them in Decisions**: Involve your child in decisions about their care, such as choosing between treatment options or setting health goals. This can help them feel more in control and motivated to follow through with treatments.
- **Respect Their Preferences**: Respect your child's preferences and comfort levels. If they are nervous about a procedure, discuss ways to make it more comfortable, such as bringing a favorite toy or listening to music.

Advocacy Beyond Healthcare Visits

Advocating for your child's health needs extends beyond healthcare visits. It involves being proactive in various aspects of their health and well-being. Here are some additional ways to advocate for your child's health:

- **Education and School**: Work with your child's school to ensure their health needs are met. This may include developing an Individualized Education Plan (IEP) for children with special needs, ensuring access to necessary medications, or creating a plan for managing chronic conditions at school.
- **Community Resources**: Utilize community resources and support networks. Many communities offer programs and services for children with specific health needs, such as support groups, therapy services, and recreational activities.
- **Healthy Lifestyle**: Promote a healthy lifestyle at home by encouraging a balanced diet, regular physical activity, adequate sleep, and stress management. These factors can significantly impact your child's overall health and well-being.
- **Preventive Care**: Emphasize the importance of preventive care, including regular check-ups, vaccinations, dental care, and vision screenings. Preventive care can help detect and address health issues early.

Dealing with Disagreements

Disagreements with healthcare providers can arise, and it's important to handle them constructively. Here are some tips for dealing with disagreements:

- **Stay Calm and Respectful**: Approach disagreements with a calm and respectful attitude. Express your concerns clearly and listen to the healthcare provider's perspective.
- **Seek a Second Opinion**: If you have significant concerns about a diagnosis or treatment plan, consider seeking a second opinion from another healthcare provider. This can provide additional insights and reassurance.
- **Use Evidence-Based Information**: Support your concerns with evidence-based information. Research reputable sources and share relevant studies or guidelines with the healthcare provider.
- **Collaborate on Solutions**: Work with the healthcare provider to find a mutually acceptable solution. This may involve compromising on

certain aspects of care or exploring alternative treatment options.

Advocacy Skills for Parents

Developing strong advocacy skills can enhance your ability to effectively communicate with healthcare providers and advocate for your child's health needs. Here are some key advocacy skills to cultivate:

- **Active Listening**: Practice active listening by paying close attention to what healthcare providers say, asking clarifying questions, and summarizing their points to ensure understanding.
- **Assertiveness**: Be assertive in expressing your child's needs and concerns. Assertiveness involves being confident and respectful in your communication, without being aggressive or passive.
- **Research Skills**: Develop your research skills to find accurate and reliable health information. Learn how to evaluate the credibility of sources and identify evidence-based recommendations.

- **Problem-Solving**: Enhance your problem-solving skills to address challenges and find effective solutions. This involves identifying the issue, generating possible solutions, evaluating options, and implementing the best course of action.
- **Emotional Intelligence**: Cultivate emotional intelligence by recognizing and managing your emotions and understanding the emotions of others. This can improve your communication and relationships with healthcare providers.

Advocating for your child's health needs is a vital aspect of parenting. By understanding your child's health, effectively communicating with healthcare providers, and building collaborative relationships, you can ensure that your child's best interests are prioritized. Remember to stay informed, be proactive, and utilize the available resources to support your child's health and well-being. Through effective advocacy, you can contribute to your child's overall health, development, and happiness.

Chapter 9: Healthy Eating and Toxin-Free Living

Healthy eating and maintaining a toxin-free environment are essential components of a holistic approach to wellness. These practices not only support the immune system but also contribute to overall physical and mental health. This chapter provides detailed guidance on nutrition tips for children and families, as well as strategies for creating a toxin-free environment at home.

Nutrition Tips for Children and Families

Proper nutrition is fundamental to a child's growth, development, and overall health. Establishing healthy eating habits early on sets the stage for a lifetime of well-being. Here, we delve into essential nutrition tips for children and families, covering various aspects of a balanced diet, important nutrients, and practical advice for encouraging healthy eating habits.

1. The Importance of a Balanced Diet

A balanced diet provides the necessary nutrients that the body needs to function optimally. These nutrients include carbohydrates, proteins, fats, vitamins, and minerals. Each plays a crucial role in supporting bodily functions, from energy production to immune defense.

- **Carbohydrates**: These are the body's primary source of energy. Opt for complex carbohydrates such as whole grains, fruits, and vegetables, which provide sustained energy and are rich in fiber.
- **Proteins**: Essential for growth and repair of tissues. Include a variety of protein sources such as lean meats, fish, eggs, beans, and nuts.
- **Fats**: Necessary for brain development and hormone production. Focus on healthy fats from sources like avocados, nuts, seeds, and olive oil.
- **Vitamins and Minerals**: Vital for various bodily functions. Ensure a diverse intake of fruits and vegetables to cover a broad spectrum of vitamins and minerals.

2. Nutrient-Rich Foods for Children

Children have specific nutritional needs due to their rapid growth and development. Incorporating nutrient-dense foods into their diet is essential for meeting these needs.

- **Dairy Products**: Provide calcium and vitamin D, important for bone health. Include milk, cheese, and yogurt.

- **Fruits and Vegetables**: Rich in vitamins, minerals, and antioxidants. Encourage a variety of colors to ensure a range of nutrients.
- **Whole Grains**: Offer fiber, B vitamins, and minerals. Examples include brown rice, whole wheat bread, and oats.
- **Lean Proteins**: Support muscle development and overall growth. Include poultry, fish, eggs, and plant-based proteins like beans and lentils.
- **Healthy Snacks**: Choose nutritious snacks such as fruit slices, yogurt, nuts, and whole-grain crackers.

3. Encouraging Healthy Eating Habits

Developing healthy eating habits in children requires a combination of education, consistency, and a positive environment. Here are strategies to promote these habits:

- **Lead by Example**: Children often mimic the behaviors of adults. Demonstrate healthy eating habits yourself to encourage them to follow suit.
- **Involve Children in Meal Preparation**: Allowing children to participate in cooking and meal planning can increase their interest in healthy foods.

- **Make Mealtimes Enjoyable**: Create a positive and relaxed atmosphere during meals. Avoid using mealtime to discipline or criticize.
- **Offer a Variety of Foods**: Introduce new foods gradually and offer a range of options to prevent picky eating.
- **Limit Processed Foods and Sugary Drinks**: Reduce the consumption of foods high in added sugars, salt, and unhealthy fats. Encourage water and milk as primary beverages.
- **Educate About Nutrition**: Teach children about the benefits of different foods and how they help the body. Use age-appropriate language and concepts.

4. Special Dietary Considerations

Some children may have specific dietary needs due to allergies, intolerances, or medical conditions. It's important to address these needs while maintaining a balanced diet.

- **Food Allergies and Intolerances**: Identify and avoid allergens, and seek alternatives to ensure nutritional adequacy. Consult with a healthcare provider or nutritionist for personalized advice.

- **Vegetarian or Vegan Diets**: Ensure sufficient intake of protein, iron, calcium, vitamin B12, and omega-3 fatty acids through plant-based sources and supplements if necessary.
- **Overweight and Obesity**: Focus on balanced meals, portion control, and physical activity rather than restrictive diets. Promote a healthy relationship with food.

5. The Role of Supplements

While a balanced diet should provide most nutrients, some situations may require supplements, especially for children with specific dietary restrictions or higher nutritional needs.

- **Vitamin D**: Important for bone health, especially in areas with limited sunlight exposure.
- **Iron**: Essential for preventing anemia, particularly in children with limited meat intake.
- **Omega-3 Fatty Acids**: Support brain development and cognitive function. Consider supplements if dietary intake is low.

6. Practical Tips for Family Meals

Creating healthy meals that the entire family enjoys can be challenging but is achievable with some practical strategies.

- **Plan Ahead**: Prepare weekly meal plans and grocery lists to ensure a variety of balanced meals.
- **Cook in Batches**: Prepare larger quantities and freeze portions for busy days.
- **Involve Everyone**: Assign age-appropriate tasks to children during meal preparation.
- **Make Healthy Swaps**: Substitute unhealthy ingredients with healthier alternatives (e.g., using Greek yogurt instead of sour cream).

Creating a Toxin-Free Environment at Home

In addition to healthy eating, creating a toxin-free environment at home is crucial for overall wellness. This involves reducing exposure to harmful chemicals and pollutants that can affect health, particularly in children who are more vulnerable to their effects.

1. Understanding Common Household Toxins

Many everyday products and materials can contain harmful substances. Awareness of these toxins and their sources is the first step in minimizing exposure.

- **Pesticides**: Found in conventional produce and household pest control products.
- **Phthalates and Parabens**: Common in personal care products such as shampoos, lotions, and cosmetics.
- **Volatile Organic Compounds (VOCs)**: Emitted from paints, cleaning products, and new furniture.
- **Heavy Metals**: Present in some old paints, plumbing materials, and certain toys.
- **Flame Retardants**: Used in furniture, electronics, and baby products.

2. Strategies for Reducing Exposure to Toxins

Implementing changes to reduce exposure to these toxins can significantly improve the health and safety of your home environment.

- **Choose Organic Produce**: Opt for organic fruits and vegetables to reduce pesticide exposure. Use the Environmental Working Group's (EWG) lists of "Dirty Dozen" and "Clean Fifteen" as guides for prioritizing organic purchases.

- **Natural Cleaning Products**: Use non-toxic, eco-friendly cleaning products or make your own using ingredients like vinegar, baking soda, and essential oils.

- **Improve Indoor Air Quality**: Increase ventilation by opening windows and using air purifiers with HEPA filters. Avoid synthetic air fresheners and candles.

- **Personal Care Products**: Select products free from phthalates, parabens, and other harmful chemicals. Look for certifications such as "USDA Organic" or "EWG Verified."

- **Safe Pest Control**: Use non-toxic methods for pest control, such as traps and natural repellents. If pesticides are necessary, follow safety guidelines and choose the least toxic options.

- **Water Quality**: Use water filters to remove contaminants from drinking water. Regularly test well water for safety.

- **Food Storage**: Avoid plastic containers and wraps that may contain BPA or phthalates. Use glass or stainless steel alternatives.

- **Reduce Flame Retardants**: Choose furniture and baby products labeled as free from added flame retardants. Regularly vacuum and dust to reduce accumulation of these chemicals.

3. Creating a Safe Nursery and Play Area

Children spend a significant amount of time in their nurseries and play areas. Ensuring these spaces are free from toxins is essential for their health.

- **Furniture and Toys**: Select items made from natural materials, such as solid wood and organic fabrics. Avoid products with chemical treatments or synthetic materials.
- **Paint and Flooring**: Use low-VOC or zero-VOC paints and finishes. Opt for natural flooring materials like hardwood, bamboo, or cork instead of carpet, which can harbor allergens and chemicals.
- **Bedding and Mattresses**: Choose organic cotton or wool bedding and mattresses free from flame retardants and other chemicals.
- **Cleaning and Maintenance**: Regularly clean and dust to minimize exposure to indoor pollutants. Use non-toxic cleaning products and wash new items before use.

4. Reducing Plastic Use

Plastics can contain harmful chemicals such as BPA, phthalates, and other endocrine disruptors. Reducing plastic use in the home can help decrease exposure to these toxins.

- **Food Containers**: Use glass, stainless steel, or silicone containers for food storage. Avoid microwaving food in plastic containers.
- **Toys and Baby Products**: Choose plastic-free options made from wood, metal, or fabric.
- **Kitchenware**: Use stainless steel or cast-iron cookware instead of non-stick pans that can release toxic fumes when overheated.
- **Household Items**: Replace plastic items with alternatives made from natural materials, such as wooden utensils and cotton bags.

5. Managing Environmental Pollutants

Environmental pollutants can also affect the indoor air quality and overall health of your home. Managing these pollutants is crucial for creating a toxin-free environment.

- **Radon**: Test your home for radon, a radioactive gas that can seep into buildings from the ground. If high levels are detected, take steps to mitigate it.
- **Lead**: If your home was built before 1978, it may contain lead-based paint. Have it inspected and, if necessary, professionally removed.
- **Asbestos**: Found in older homes, asbestos can be harmful when disturbed. If you suspect its presence, hire a professional to handle it.
- **Pesticides and Herbicides**: Limit the use of chemical pesticides and herbicides in your garden. Opt for organic gardening methods and natural pest control solutions.

6. Educating and Involving the Family

Creating a toxin-free environment is a collective effort that involves educating and involving all family members. Encourage everyone to adopt and maintain healthy practices.

- **Education**: Teach children about the importance of a healthy environment and how to make safe choices. Explain why certain products are avoided and the benefits of natural alternatives.

- **Involvement**: Include family members in the process of choosing non-toxic products and implementing changes. Foster a sense of responsibility and teamwork.
- **Consistency**: Consistently follow and reinforce toxin-free practices to create lasting habits and a healthier home environment.

7. Long-Term Benefits of a Toxin-Free Lifestyle

Adopting a toxin-free lifestyle has numerous long-term benefits for both children and adults. These benefits extend beyond immediate health improvements and contribute to overall well-being.

- **Reduced Risk of Chronic Diseases**: Minimizing exposure to harmful chemicals can lower the risk of developing chronic conditions such as asthma, allergies, and certain cancers.
- **Enhanced Immune Function**: A toxin-free environment supports the immune system, helping the body better defend against illnesses and infections.
- **Improved Mental Health**: Reducing exposure to environmental toxins can positively impact mental health, reducing stress and improving cognitive function.

- **Sustainable Living**: Choosing non-toxic, eco-friendly products supports sustainable living practices, benefiting the environment and future generations.

Healthy eating and maintaining a toxin-free environment are integral components of a holistic approach to wellness. By focusing on nutrient-rich foods and reducing exposure to harmful chemicals, you can create a healthier, safer, and more supportive environment for your family. The benefits of these practices extend beyond physical health, fostering a sense of well-being and resilience that can last a lifetime.

Chapter 10: Making Informed Healthcare Decisions

Understanding Risks and Benefits of Vaccination

In the realm of healthcare, making informed decisions is paramount, especially when it comes to vaccination. Vaccines are one of the most significant medical advancements in human history, responsible for eradicating or controlling many infectious diseases that once caused widespread morbidity and mortality. However, like all medical interventions, vaccines come with their own set of risks and benefits. Understanding these risks and benefits is crucial for making informed healthcare decisions for yourself and your family.

The Benefits of Vaccination

1. **Prevention of Disease:** The primary benefit of vaccination is the prevention of infectious diseases. Vaccines have been instrumental in reducing the incidence of diseases such as measles, polio, and whooping cough. For example, the smallpox vaccine led to the eradication of smallpox worldwide, saving countless lives and preventing suffering.

2. **Herd Immunity:** Vaccination not only protects the individual who receives the vaccine but also contributes to herd immunity. Herd immunity occurs when a significant portion of a population becomes immune to a disease, thereby providing indirect protection to those who are not immune, such as newborns, the elderly, or individuals with compromised immune systems. This community-level protection is crucial in preventing outbreaks of contagious diseases.

3. **Reduction in Healthcare Costs:** Preventing disease through vaccination reduces the overall burden on the healthcare system. Vaccinated individuals are less likely to require medical treatment, hospitalization, or long-term care due to vaccine-preventable diseases. This translates into significant cost savings for both individuals and healthcare systems.

4. **Improved Quality of Life:** By preventing serious illnesses, vaccines contribute to an improved quality of life. Children who are vaccinated are less likely to miss school due to illness, and parents are less likely to miss work to care for sick children. Additionally, preventing diseases like HPV can reduce the risk of certain cancers, further enhancing long-term health outcomes.

The Risks of Vaccination

1. **Common Side Effects:** Like any medical intervention, vaccines can cause side effects. The most common side effects are mild and temporary, such as pain at the injection site, low-grade fever, and mild rash. These side effects are generally short-lived and resolve on their own without requiring medical treatment.

2. **Rare Adverse Reactions:** While serious adverse reactions to vaccines are rare, they can occur. These may include severe allergic reactions (anaphylaxis), high fever, or febrile seizures. It is important to note that the risk of serious adverse reactions is much lower than the risk of complications from the diseases that vaccines prevent.

3. **Myths and Misconceptions:** Misinformation about vaccines can contribute to fear and hesitancy. Common myths, such as the belief that vaccines cause autism, have been thoroughly debunked by extensive research. However, these myths persist and can influence individuals' perceptions of vaccine risks.

Evaluating the Risk-Benefit Balance

When making healthcare decisions, it is essential to evaluate the risk-benefit balance. This involves comparing the risks associated with vaccination to the risks of not vaccinating and potentially contracting the disease. Here are some key considerations:

1. **Disease Severity and Complications:** Many vaccine-preventable diseases can cause severe illness, long-term complications, or death. For example, measles can lead to encephalitis (brain swelling) and pneumonia, while pertussis (whooping cough) can cause severe respiratory distress, particularly in infants. The risks of these complications far outweigh the risks of mild vaccine side effects.

2. **Vaccine Safety Monitoring:** Vaccines undergo rigorous testing in clinical trials to assess their safety and efficacy before being approved for public use. Once approved, vaccines continue to be monitored through robust surveillance systems to identify and investigate any potential safety concerns. This ongoing monitoring ensures that vaccines remain safe and effective for the population.

3. **Individual Health Considerations:** It is important to consider individual health conditions and risk factors when making vaccination decisions. For example, individuals with certain medical conditions may need to avoid specific vaccines or follow modified vaccination schedules. Consulting with a healthcare provider can help determine the best approach based on individual health needs.

Addressing Common Concerns and Questions

Despite the overwhelming evidence supporting the safety and efficacy of vaccines, many people have concerns and questions about vaccination. Addressing these concerns with accurate information and empathy is crucial for building trust and promoting informed healthcare decisions.

1. **Are Vaccines Safe?** Vaccines are among the safest medical interventions available. Before approval, vaccines undergo rigorous testing in clinical trials to evaluate their safety and efficacy. Once approved, vaccines continue to be monitored for safety through extensive surveillance systems. The benefits of vaccination

in preventing serious diseases far outweigh the risks of rare adverse reactions.

2. **Do Vaccines Cause Autism?** The claim that vaccines cause autism originated from a 1998 study that has since been thoroughly discredited and retracted. Extensive research involving millions of children has found no link between vaccines and autism. Major health organizations, including the Centers for Disease Control and Prevention (CDC) and the World Health Organization (WHO), affirm that vaccines do not cause autism.

3. **Can Vaccines Overwhelm the Immune System?** The immune system is capable of handling multiple vaccines at once. Vaccines contain antigens, which are substances that stimulate the immune response. The number of antigens in vaccines is a tiny fraction of what the immune system encounters daily. Scientific evidence shows that receiving multiple vaccines simultaneously does not overwhelm the immune system.

4. **What About Vaccine Ingredients?** Some people are concerned about the ingredients in vaccines, such as preservatives, adjuvants, and stabilizers. These ingredients are used to ensure the safety

and effectiveness of vaccines. For example, thimerosal, a mercury-based preservative, has been removed from most vaccines, and extensive research has shown it to be safe. Vaccine ingredients are present in very small amounts and are rigorously tested for safety.

5. **Why Do Some Vaccines Require Multiple Doses?** Some vaccines require multiple doses to provide long-lasting immunity. The first dose helps the immune system recognize the pathogen, and subsequent doses strengthen and prolong the immune response. This approach ensures optimal protection against the disease. Booster doses may also be needed to maintain immunity over time.

6. **Can Natural Immunity Replace Vaccination?** Natural immunity occurs when a person becomes immune to a disease after being infected and recovering from it. While natural immunity can provide protection, it often comes at a high cost, including severe illness, complications, and potential death. Vaccination provides immunity without the risks associated with natural infection.

7. **What If My Child Misses a Vaccination?** If your child misses a scheduled vaccination, consult with your healthcare provider to determine the best

course of action. Most vaccines can be given on a catch-up schedule to ensure your child is protected. It is important to complete the full vaccination series to achieve optimal immunity.

8. **Are Vaccines Necessary If a Disease Is Rare?** Vaccines remain necessary even if a disease is rare in your community. Vaccination helps prevent the resurgence of diseases that are currently under control. Additionally, global travel can introduce diseases from other regions, making vaccination an essential tool for protecting public health.

Making informed healthcare decisions about vaccination requires a thorough understanding of the risks and benefits. Vaccines are a safe and effective way to prevent serious diseases, protect public health, and improve the quality of life. While vaccines can cause mild side effects and rare adverse reactions, the risks of vaccine-preventable diseases far outweigh these risks.

Addressing common concerns and questions with accurate information and empathy is crucial for building trust and promoting informed healthcare decisions. By understanding the science behind vaccines, consulting with healthcare providers, and considering individual health needs, parents can make the best decisions for their children's health and well-being.

Informed decision-making is the cornerstone of vaccine-friendly parenting. By educating yourself about vaccines and their role in preventing disease, you can confidently navigate the complex world of healthcare and ensure the health and safety of your family. Remember, vaccination is not just a personal choice; it is a collective responsibility that contributes to the health and well-being of the entire community.

In the end, the goal of vaccination is to create a healthier, safer world for everyone. By making informed healthcare decisions, you are playing a crucial role in achieving this goal and building a stronger, healthier future for your family and community.

Conclusion

As we come to the end of "A Vaccine-Friendly Guide for Parenting: A Practical Approach for Building Stronger Families through Informed Wellness, and Unlocking Health Potential," it is essential to reflect on the key principles of vaccine-friendly parenting and look ahead to how we can sustain health and wellness in our families and communities. This conclusion aims to reinforce the concepts discussed throughout the book and provide a roadmap for maintaining a holistic approach to health.

Recap of Vaccine-Friendly Parenting Principles

Throughout this book, we have explored various aspects of vaccine-friendly parenting. These principles are designed to empower you with the knowledge and confidence needed to make informed health decisions for your family. Let's recap the core principles of vaccine-friendly parenting:

1. **Informed Decision-Making**: The foundation of vaccine-friendly parenting is informed decision-making. This involves educating yourself about vaccines, understanding their benefits and risks, and making decisions based on accurate,

evidence-based information. Informed parents are better equipped to navigate the complex landscape of vaccination and health care.

2. **Building Trust with Healthcare Providers**: A strong, trusting relationship with your healthcare providers is crucial. Open communication with pediatricians, family doctors, and nurses allows for a collaborative approach to your child's health. Trust is built through respectful dialogue, asking questions, and seeking professional guidance.

3. **Understanding the Science of Vaccines**: Knowledge of how vaccines work and their role in preventing disease is essential. Vaccines stimulate the immune system to recognize and fight pathogens without causing the disease itself. Understanding this process helps demystify vaccines and underscores their importance in protecting public health.

4. **Addressing Concerns and Misconceptions**: Vaccine-friendly parenting involves addressing concerns and debunking myths about vaccines. By confronting misinformation with evidence-based explanations, you can alleviate fears and build confidence in the vaccination process. Recognizing that concerns often stem from

genuine care for children's well-being is key to empathetic communication.

5. **Holistic Health and Wellness**: Vaccines are a vital part of preventive health care, but they are not the only factor in maintaining good health. A holistic approach to wellness includes nutrition, physical activity, mental health, and a supportive environment. By integrating these elements, you create a comprehensive health plan for your family.

6. **Community and Herd Immunity**: Understanding the concept of herd immunity highlights the collective responsibility of vaccination. Vaccinating your child not only protects them but also contributes to the health of the community, particularly those who cannot be vaccinated for medical reasons. This sense of collective responsibility fosters a healthier society.

By adhering to these principles, you can navigate the challenges of parenting with confidence and a focus on informed wellness. Your role as a parent is pivotal in ensuring the health and safety of your child and contributing to the broader goal of public health.

Looking Ahead: Sustaining Health and Wellness

As we look ahead, it is important to consider how we can sustain health and wellness beyond the scope of vaccination. The principles discussed in this book provide a solid foundation, but maintaining health is an ongoing journey that requires commitment and adaptability. Here are some strategies for sustaining health and wellness in your family and community:

1. **Stay Informed**: Health recommendations and scientific understanding continue to evolve. Staying informed about the latest research and guidelines is crucial for making up-to-date decisions. Subscribe to reputable health news sources, attend seminars, and engage with community health initiatives to keep your knowledge current.

2. **Promote Healthy Habits**: Encourage and model healthy habits in your family. A balanced diet rich in fruits, vegetables, whole grains, and lean proteins supports overall health. Regular physical activity, adequate sleep, and mental health care are equally important. These habits not only boost the immune system but also contribute to long-term well-being.

3. **Foster Open Communication**: Maintain open lines of communication with your children about health and wellness. Educate them about the

importance of vaccines and other preventive measures. By fostering a culture of openness and curiosity, you empower your children to take an active role in their health.

4. **Engage with Your Community**: Community engagement plays a significant role in sustaining health and wellness. Participate in local health initiatives, support public health campaigns, and advocate for policies that promote access to vaccines and healthcare services. By being an active member of your community, you contribute to a healthier environment for everyone.

5. **Monitor and Manage Health**: Regular health check-ups are essential for early detection and management of potential health issues. Follow recommended vaccination schedules, attend routine medical appointments, and be vigilant about any changes in your family's health. Proactive health management ensures that you can address issues promptly and maintain optimal wellness.

6. **Educate and Advocate**: Use your knowledge to educate others about the importance of vaccines and informed wellness. Share reliable information with friends, family, and community members.

Advocacy can take many forms, from participating in school health programs to engaging in public discussions about health policies. Your voice can make a difference in promoting health literacy and vaccine acceptance.

7. **Prepare for Emergencies**: Health emergencies, such as outbreaks of vaccine-preventable diseases, can arise unexpectedly. Having a plan in place ensures that you are prepared to respond effectively. This includes keeping vaccination records up to date, knowing the signs and symptoms of diseases, and having access to medical care when needed.

8. **Adapt to New Challenges**: The health landscape is constantly changing, with new challenges and opportunities emerging. Being adaptable and resilient in the face of change is crucial for sustaining wellness. Whether it's responding to new vaccine recommendations or adjusting health practices in response to emerging threats, flexibility is key.

In conclusion, vaccine-friendly parenting is about more than just following a vaccination schedule. It is a holistic approach that encompasses informed decision-making, building trust with healthcare providers, understanding the science, addressing concerns, promoting overall wellness, and engaging with the community. By adhering to these principles and looking ahead with a proactive mindset, you can ensure the health and well-being of your family and contribute to a healthier society.

Thank you for embarking on this journey of informed wellness with us. We hope that this book has provided you with valuable insights and practical tools to navigate the complexities of parenting and health care. Remember, your role as a parent is vital in shaping the future health of your child and community. Together, we can build stronger families through informed wellness and unlock the full potential of health for generations to come.

I HAVE A REQUEST

Dear Reader,

Thank you for your purchase! We hope you enjoyed the book. We would greatly appreciate it if you could leave an honest review.

Your honest feedback is essential for our growth and helps us understand what you value most. By sharing your thoughts, you not only help other readers make informed choices but also increase the visibility of this book.

Your words can inspire and guide others, creating a community built on shared insights and connections. Let's celebrate meaningful communication and the beauty of heartfelt expressions together.

Thank you!